Weight Loss Success Using Six Sigma

Sterling Thompson

National Library of Canada Cataloguing in Publication

Thompson, Sterling
     Weight loss success using six sigma / Sterling Thompson.

ISBN 1-55395-437-8

     1. Weight loss. 2. Six Sigma (Quality control standard)
I. Title.

RM222.2.T4852 2003   613.2'5   C2002-906066-4

TRAFFORD

This book was published *on-demand* in cooperation with Trafford Publishing.
On-demand publishing is a unique process and service of making a book available for retail sale to the public taking advantage of on-demand manufacturing and Internet marketing. **On-demand publishing** includes promotions, retail sales, manufacturing, order fulfilment, accounting and collecting royalties on behalf of the author.

Suite 6E, 2333 Government St., Victoria, B.C. V8T 4P4, CANADA
Phone   250-383-6864   Toll-free 1-888-232-4444 (Canada & US)
Fax   250-383-6804   E-mail   sales@trafford.com
Web site www.trafford.com   TRAFFORD PUBLISHING IS A DIVISION OF TRAFFORD HOLDINGS LTD.
Trafford Catalogue #02-1152   www.trafford.com/robots/02-1152.html

10   9   8   7   6   5   4   3

Acknowledgments

I wish to thank Sherri Snyder for her excellent copy editing of this book. She spent many hours reviewing and improving the manuscript. This would not have been possible without her work.

I also would like to thank my wife Lana for her help and patience as I put this book together. My wife was also a great help in proofreading the book for me.

Thank you both for all of your help.

Supplemental Materials

This book will discuss using data tables and charts. Visit my website at www.SixSigmaWeightLoss.com where blank data tables and charts are available for download.

Table of Contents

My Reason for Writing This Book

In the fall of 2001, I was given a great opportunity by my employer to be trained in the Six Sigma business improvement program. Six Sigma was designed for businesses to improve their effectiveness. While I was sitting in training, I was thinking about what is one of the most difficult things to do. Since they fed us extremely well at training and I felt my clothes getting tighter, I thought of personal weight loss. An entire industry is dedicated to weight loss. It is not only difficult to lose weight, but it is even more difficult to keep the weight off once a person loses it.

Six Sigma is designed not only to help a person make improvements but also to sustain what one has done. Six Sigma programs call it "Sustain the Gain." It is probably more appropriate to call it "Sustain the Loss" for this book's purpose.

Six Sigma training is done in four weeks where a person trains for one week a month for four months. My training was in September, October, November, and December.

My significant weight gain was the result of the fantastic meals during training. The first week alone I gained 5 pounds. Knowing this, I cut back on desserts and snacks the next 3 weeks of training, and I only added an additional 5 pounds. So training increased not only my knowledge but also my waistline by 10 pounds.

I had another thing going against me; the last week of training was between Thanksgiving and Christmas. This time of the year is always a good time to add even more weight.

On January 2, the reality of my extra weight became obvious. I put on my clothes for work. I was wearing a thick flannel shirt. The shirt was no problem getting on, but I barely got my pants zipped. That was the time I decided that I must do something about my weight. I'm too cheap to buy bigger sized clothes, so the weight had to go.

I needed a tangible reward for my effort besides looking and feeling better in my clothes, however. Then I remembered that I had received a $100 in Christmas money that I had not yet spent, and I knew the coming summer, my family was going to a place where a round of golf is $100. Therefore, I made a deal with myself. If I lose 20 pounds by the beginning of June, I would play a round of golf using that $100. If I did not lose it, I would not get to play golf.

With thoughts of summer, I had my goal. I just needed a way to reach this goal. This was the time where I thought back to my experiences while training on Six Sigma. This program would be perfect to use to reach my goal. I would use the Six Sigma philosophy to lose weight and keep it off.

Although the original intent of Six Sigma is not a diet plan, it is a method to help with whatever diet plan one is following. It can also help sustain the accomplishment of the weight already lost. By sustaining the weight loss, the cycle of losing weight will not have to be endured again.

I am writing this book to share my experience so that others may be able to use my experience to help reach their weight loss goals. If Six Sigma is utilized in one's personal life, he/she can say, "I not only know about Six Sigma, but I am also living it."

Explanation of Six Sigma

Before diving into how Six Sigma can be used in weight loss, a quick review of Six Sigma is necessary. Six Sigma is a business improvement program that was originally conceptualized in the 1980's by Motorola. Companies began to use the program with great success. Some of the additional companies to embrace Six Sigma include General Electric, Caterpillar, and The Dow Chemical Company. This program is not any new statistic or control chart system because Six Sigma took methods and tools already developed by others and created a program that tied these pieces into one comprehensive program.

Six Sigma has people pulled out of their normal duties and has these people trained on the Six Sigma methodology. Once people are trained, they lead projects to improve a company process. Each trained person is called a Black Belt who leads a project team through a project to address whatever process is given to them.

This improvement program is very data driven. Its philosophy is if something cannot be measured, it cannot be improved. There are no personal subjective feelings about how a process is doing. Data has to be gathered to prove any feelings or theories.

The Six Sigma process is broken up into 4 main phases. The phases are Measure, Analyze, Improve, and Control. This methodology takes a problem or process and fixes the problem or process continually.

The Measure Phase of a project comes up with a way of measuring how the process is doing. After figuring out a way to measure the process, the project team must collect the data to find out how the process is doing.

The Analyze Phase of the project is where one tries to figure out why the process is where it is. The project team digs deep to find the root cause of the problems. Once it gets by the symptoms, it can get to the real causes of the problem.

The Improve Phase is the time where the project team comes up with a plan to eliminate these root causes. Once the root causes are eliminated, the problem goes away and the process has a big improvement.

The Control Phase is different from the rest of the programs of the month. The Control Phase documents the improvement plan and the new process. It also identifies whoever is responsible to keep the process going after project team disbands. This person must take ownership of the new process and make sure the process is followed. The Control Phase also defines a way of measuring the new process to make sure the improvements stick and not slowly, or quickly, go away.

This program is based on getting data and then analyzing it. Weight loss lends itself quite well to Six Sigma since it is easily measured. Consequently, the philosophy of Six Sigma's measuring and improving is a concrete, objective way to lose weight. Six Sigma and weight loss have a workable connection that will accomplish losing those unwanted, unhealthy pounds.

My Personal Weight History

Perhaps some other background information is needed about my personal weight history. I found my eighth grade height and weight on a strip of paper in my eighth grade report card. I was 5'9" and 155 pounds. For the basketball team's weigh in during my sophomore year of high school, I was 5'9" and 165 pounds. This was probably the peak of my physical condition. The following year, I was still 5'9," but I was 175 pounds. After this point, I continued at my height of 5'9," and my weight fluctuated between 180 pounds and 200 pounds.

Four years before I went on my Six Sigma diet, I did the Weight Watchers Points diet with my wife. I was able to go from 195 pounds down to 175 pounds. Then like all casual dieters, I stopped paying close attention to my weight. I first said that I would stay between 175 and 180 pounds. Once I went over 180 pounds, I told myself to watch it and get back down to 180 pounds. I did not go over 185 pounds, but I never got back to 180 pounds.

Then I was chosen to take the Black Belt training of Six Sigma. During that four months of training, I increased my weight to 195 pounds, and my clothes were not fitting well at all. I was very uncomfortable. The meals at these training sessions were unbelievably good, which did not help the tight clothes problem. These first weight measurements were done with clothes on. All weight measurements that follow were done without clothes, so there is about a 4 pound difference in the weight measurements. In other words, instead of being 195 pounds, I actually weighed 191 pounds.

Losing Weight Using Six Sigma

Although Six Sigma is not a diet plan, it complements the diet plan that one is using. I learned a lot about how I can lose weight through moderation and substitution, and I also learned how my body reacted to food. Of course, checking out one's diet plan with his/her physician before starting is important.

My documenting my weight loss using Six Sigma may prove to be a helpful guide for anyone who is serious about losing weight and keeping it off. By going through my weight loss experience, one should be able to develop how to apply Six Sigma to his/her own personal weight loss system.

This book will discuss using data tables and charts. Visit my website at www.SixSigmaWeightLoss.com where blank data tables and charts are available for download.

The Measure Phase

Of course, the first task of Six Sigma is to measure one's weight. This can be done using a scale. The better the scale, the more accurate the weight measurement will be although the scale does not have to be great. The scale I used would regularly be off by 1½ pounds. There will always be errors in the scale readings. In the long run, a 2 pound reading error will not matter much if one is losing 20 pounds or more.

The other thing I did was to take my weight measurement at the same time each day and with the same level of clothing. Body weight will go up and down throughout the day by multiple pounds. A glass of water temporary adds 1 pound of weight. So if a person weighs at the same time each day, he/she will minimize the fluctuations between the weight readings.

Also clothes can change weight readings. My work clothes with shoes weigh about 4 pounds. If I started my weight measurements in the winter with heavy clothes and then went to summer and started weighing in shorts, I would lose a pound or two just because of the clothes.

As a result, to help minimize the weight reading differences, I would weigh myself each morning when I got up. I also weighed without any clothes to take the clothes weight variance totally out of play.

Now a person does not have to weigh like I did. On my previous diet, I weighed at work around 9:00 in the morning. I weighed on a certified shipping scale so that I had an accurate scale reading, but I added fluctuations in the weight measurements due to clothes and any morning eating extras, like doughnuts.

How often does a person weigh? Most diets talk about weighing once a week. This is because one's weight will fluctuate during the week. This is all true, but I found waiting the whole week gave me no feedback on how I was doing or what I was doing that was affecting my weight. I weighed every day. I was able to find out the things that worked for me. My weight would go up and down and all around during the week; but as I built my weight readings, I started to see patterns and was able to improve my weight loss program. Therefore, I weighed each day and understood that it would go up and down each day. This information was valuable in the Analyze Phase.

After getting the scale and weighing at the same time each day, I needed to record the numbers. I used a computer spreadsheet to record my weight measurements. I set up a table that had the date, day of the week, and weight measurement. It turned out that the day of the week was important in my weight analysis. I also had the spreadsheet do two calculations. The first was to compare today's weight to yesterday's weight. The other calculation was to compare today's weight to last week's weight on the same day of the week.

The basic spreadsheet looked like this

Date	Day of Week	Weight (lb)	Previous Day Change	Previous Week Change
14-Dec-01	Friday	**188.0**		
15-Dec-01	Saturday	188.5	0.5	
16-Dec-01	Sunday	187.0	(1.5)	
17-Dec-01	Monday	189.5	2.5	
18-Dec-01	Tuesday	187.0	(2.5)	
19-Dec-01	Wednesday	187.0	0.0	
20-Dec-01	Thursday	185.5	(1.5)	
21-Dec-01	Friday	**186.5**	**1.0**	**(1.5)**
22-Dec-01	Saturday	186.5	0.0	(2.0)
23-Dec-01	Sunday	187.0	0.5	0.0
24-Dec-01	Monday	188.5	1.5	(1.0)
25-Dec-01	Tuesday	188.5	0.0	1.5
26-Dec-01	Wednesday	188.5	0.0	1.5
27-Dec-01	Thursday	186.0	(2.5)	0.5
28-Dec 01	Friday	**188.5**	**2.5**	**2.0**

If a computer spreadsheet to record measurements is not available, write it down on a piece of paper. Then instead of the spreadsheet making the weight comparison calculations, one just has to manually make the calculation by subtracting today's weight from yesterday's weight and from the previous week's weight.

To make weight comparisons easier, a person should probably record weight to the nearest pound or ½ pound. Therefore, if the digital scale says one's weight is 178.4 pounds, he/she would record 178.0 pounds if rounding to the nearest pound, or he/she would record 178.5 pounds if rounding to the nearest ½ pound.

One does not get any value by trying to weigh more accurately. The truth is the scale cannot accurately weigh a person that well. I was pushing the accuracy of my readings by recording to the ½ pound since I knew my scale could be off by 1½ pounds.

There were two other things that I added to my computer spreadsheet. First, I added a column for comments. This was helpful when I started to analyze my information. For example, I had multiple birthday dinners to go to in March. I am not one to turn down cake and ice cream, so I did not lose weight during March. I could write "birthday dinner" in the comment's column to help explain why the weight measurements went the way they did. In my case, the weight stayed the same. Conversely, one can also add good things like going to an aerobics class. I could write in "basketball" for my Wednesday comment because I played basketball on most Wednesday nights.

The other bit of information I added to the computer spreadsheet was my weight goal line. If a person does not have an ultimate goal along with intermediate goals, it makes it quite difficult to achieve what he/she wants. How can one get to where he/she is going without first knowing where he/she is going?

In my case, I set a goal of reaching 168 pounds by the time of our family vacation to the beach. Looking good in the bathing suit is most likely many people's goal. I set this goal at the start of the year when I weighed 188 pounds. From my previous dieting experience, I knew a person could sustain a long-term weight loss of 1 to 2 pounds a week.

At first, I set high hopes of losing 1½ pounds a week. For the first 2 months, I was able to maintain this weight loss level. Then March hit, and I got away from this goal. I went back to my chart and added a goal of losing 1 pound each week. This rate would still get me to my overall goal weight. I was then able to maintain the 1 pound per week weight loss without getting discouraged.

I chose 168 pounds because this was about what I weighed in high school. A person has to pick a goal weight of where to stop. If one does not, he/she will never be able to get to the Control Phase of Six Sigma.

Getting to the goal weight will not be a quick endeavor. I wanted to lose 20 pounds, and it almost took me a half a year. One may need to go a year or even more. One should not get discouraged; he/she will be able to see progress. Even though it may seem slow, the results will be worth it.

Once the ending weight goal has been determined, intermediate goals are essential. I chose to have a weekly goal. Every Friday was my intermediate goal weigh day. I would compare my Friday weight to my goal for the week. This would let me know how I was doing.

I also ended up having two goal weights. At first I had a goal to lose 1½ pounds a week. I then added a goal of losing 1 pound a week. I started the 1 pound a week back at the beginning of my measurements.

The computer spreadsheet looked like this:

Date	Day of Week	Weight (lb)	Previous Day Change	Previous Week Change	Comments	1½ Pound Loss Goal	1 Pound Loss Goal
1-Jan-02	Tue	189.5	1.5	1.0	Started $100 Challenge		
2-Jan-02	Wed	191.0	1.5	2.5			
3-Jan-02	Thu	189.0	(2.0)	3.0			
4-Jan-02	Fri	**189.5**	**0.5**	**1.0**		**188**	**188**
5-Jan-02	Sat	188.0	(1.5)	(1.0)			
6-Jan-02	Sun	188.5	0.5	(0.5)			
7-Jan-02	Mon	188.0	(0.5)	0.0			
8-Jan-02	Tue	187.0	(1.0)	(2.5)			
9-Jan-02	Wed	186.0	(1.0)	(5.0)	Basketball		
10-Jan-02	Thu	185.5	(0.5)	(3.5)			
11-Jan-02	Fri	**187.0**	**1.5**	**(2.5)**		**186.5**	**187**
12-Jan-02	Sat	186.0	(1.0)	(2.0)			
13-Jan-02	Sun	186.5	0.5	(2.0)			
14-Jan-02	Mon	186.0	(0.5)	(2.0)			
15-Jan-02	Tue	184.0	(2.0)	(3.0)			
16-Jan-02	Wed	184.5	0.5	(1.5)	Basketball		
17-Jan-02	Thu	183.5	(1.0)	(2.0)			
18-Jan-02	Fri	**185.0**	**1.5**	**(2.0)**		**185**	**186**

The last thing I did with the computer spreadsheet was to create a graph of this information. The computer spreadsheet really is convenient on graphing since it automatically updates the information, but a computer spreadsheet to graph the information is not mandatory because basic graph paper will clearly show the same results.

The graph is a time graph of the weight. The date is used to mark the bottom of the graph or X-axis. The side of the graph or Y-axis is the weight. The weight is used to mark where the person is on the graph. So each day a weight point is added to the graph. Then one can connect a line from the previous day's weight to today's weight. The resulting plot will be jerky with the line going up and down and all over the place; but if one is losing weight, he/she will see a downward trend.

To help see how one is doing, just add a straight line of how much one is planning to lose each week. I ended up with 2 goal lines with one for 1½ pounds per week and one for 1 pound per week. Both of the lines started at my starting date of the diet, and they diverged out as time went on.

One can make the goal line by adding dots at the intermediate goal weight from the weight table and plot them on the graph. Then one should then be able to connect the points with a straight line. In my case, I had two goal lines, and my weight basically stayed at or between the two lines.

These goal lines ended up being very important to me. When I would get discouraged, I could look at the chart to see that I was really losing weight. Conversely, the goal lines would signal to me that things are not going as well as I hoped and that I needed to make a change in my plan to get me back on track.

My weight chart ended up looking like this:

January to April Weight Chart

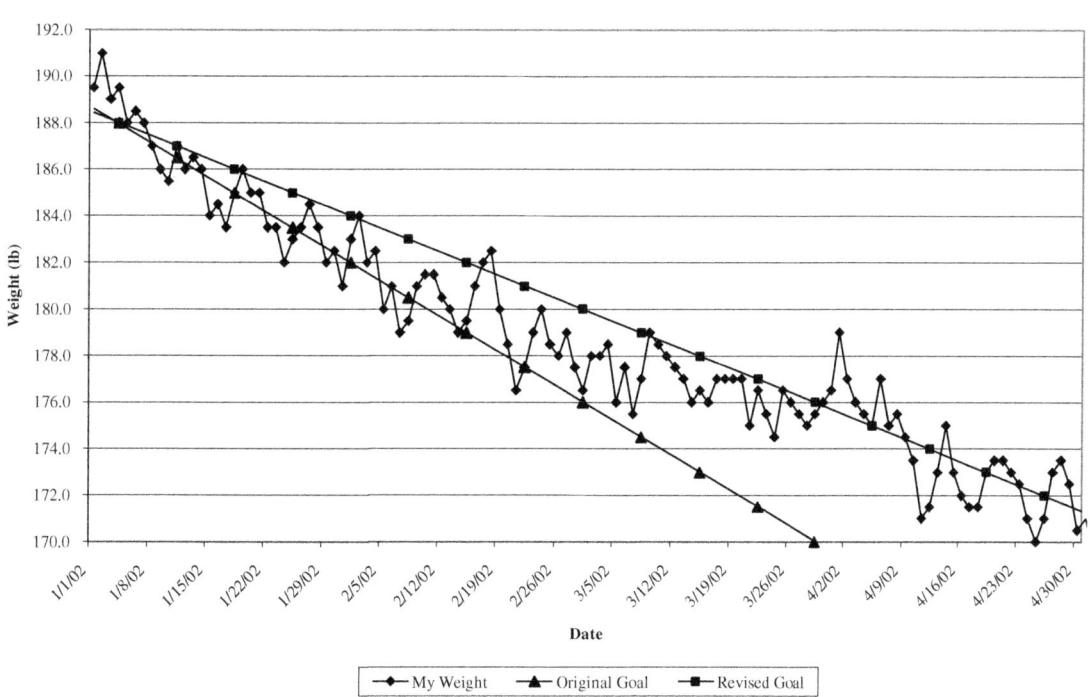

Having the tools to measure one's weight and tracking it against one's goal complete the Measure Phase of Six Sigma. The person is measuring where he/she is and has meaningful data and a meaningful way of visualizing the data. The next parts of Six Sigma are the Analyze and Improve Phases.

The Analyze and Improve Phases

As I stated at the beginning of this book, this is not a diet plan. The use of Six Sigma is to be a complement to whatever diet plan one is using.

Due to my previous dieting, I basically knew what I needed to do to lose weight. I did the following things:

1) I cut out nighttime snacking. I previously enjoyed a can of Mountain Dew and popcorn or other snack food while watching television. I cut this out. Instead, I substituted a bottle of water and a Tootsie Pop sucker. This way I was able to tell my stomach it was full with the water and with the sugar from the sucker. I think this also helped to keep my body's metabolism up at night.

2) I ate in moderation. I stopped getting seconds on food, only one plate of food instead of two. That is tough to do, so sometimes I would get a small first helping and then get a small second helping. Together they add up to just one serving.

3) I substituted foods especially when eating out. For instance at Wendy's, I would get the five piece chicken nuggets instead of the single hamburger with cheese. If I wanted the taste of hamburger, I would get the junior instead of the single. This was difficult to do when I was hungry, but I discovered I could satisfy my urge with the smaller hamburger.

This is basically what I did to lose weight. One's diet plan will not be like mine because it was tailored to my personal behaviors and body responses. There are many diet plans available to follow. Whatever diet plan is chosen will be compatible with the methods described in this book, and these methods will help that diet plan work.

Using this Six Sigma methodology will help gauge how a person is doing. It will give better information of where one is and the direction of where he/she is going. As the diet process goes along, one will be able to find out what is working, what is not working, and the impact of any eating events like my rash of birthday parties with cake and ice cream. After finding out what works, continue doing it and stop doing the things that do not work.

Based upon this information, one should be able to go back and make changes to the diet plan to help it work better. One keeps making improvements as he/she goes along. One can never stop measuring, analyzing, and improving until the goal is reached. Then one will get to enjoy the Control Phase of Six Sigma.

So the question is how do I analyze this data I am collecting each day? At first there is not enough data to see any trends or provide any useful data to analyze. The first couple of weeks, one just does the diet and records the weight on the table and chart. Hopefully, some pounds are being lost during this time. This is usually the easiest time to lose weight. If this is not happening, then one may want to make adjustments to or change the diet plan.

When one has collected data for a couple of weeks, he/she can start looking at the data. When I did my diet, I had the luxury of putting the data into a statistical computer package that did the comparisons for me. Based upon what I found out, I will illustrate how one can do this without any computers. I will show how I analyzed my readings, which should give a constructive guide of how the data can be analyzed.

My Weight Data for January

Date	Day of Week	Weight (lb)	Previous Day Change	Previous Week Change	1½ Pound Loss Goal
1-Jan-02	Tuesday	189.5	1.5	1.0	
2-Jan-02	Wednesday	191.0	1.5	2.5	
3-Jan-02	Thursday	189.0	(2.0)	3.0	
4-Jan-02	Friday	**189.5**	**0.5**	**1.0**	**188**
5-Jan-02	Saturday	188.0	(1.5)	(1.0)	
6-Jan-02	Sunday	188.5	0.5	(0.5)	
7-Jan-02	Monday	188.0	(0.5)	0.0	
8-Jan-02	Tuesday	187.0	(1.0)	(2.5)	
9-Jan-02	Wednesday	186.0	(1.0)	(5.0)	
10-Jan-02	Thursday	185.5	(0.5)	(3.5)	
11-Jan-02	Friday	**187.0**	**1.5**	**(2.5)**	**186.5**
12-Jan-02	Saturday	186.0	(1.0)	(2.0)	
13-Jan-02	Sunday	186.5	0.5	(2.0)	
14-Jan-02	Monday	186.0	(0.5)	(2.0)	
15-Jan-02	Tuesday	184.0	(2.0)	(3.0)	
16-Jan-02	Wednesday	184.5	0.5	(1.5)	
17-Jan-02	Thursday	183.5	(1.0)	(2.0)	
18-Jan-02	Friday	**185.0**	**1.5**	**(2.0)**	**185**
19-Jan-02	Saturday	186.0	1.0	0.0	
20-Jan-02	Sunday	185.0	(1.0)	(1.5)	
21-Jan-02	Monday	185.0	0.0	(1.0)	
22-Jan-02	Tuesday	183.5	(1.5)	(0.5)	
23-Jan-02	Wednesday	183.5	0.0	(1.0)	
24-Jan-02	Thursday	182.0	(1.5)	(1.5)	
25-Jan-02	Friday	**183.0**	**1.0**	**(2.0)**	**183.5**
26-Jan-02	Saturday	183.5	0.5	(2.5)	
27-Jan-02	Sunday	184.5	1.0	(0.5)	
28-Jan-02	Monday	183.5	(1.0)	(1.5)	
29-Jan-02	Tuesday	182.0	(1.5)	(1.5)	
30-Jan-02	Wednesday	182.5	0.5	(1.0)	
31-Jan-02	Thursday	181.0	(1.5)	(1.0)	
1-Feb-02	Friday	**183.0**	**2.0**	**0.0**	**182**

I had a goal line of losing 1½ pounds a week. I was able to meet this goal on most Fridays. From looking at the data, here are a few things I noticed:

1)   My week to week weight loss looked real good. Each day I was either at the same weight or lower weight than that day the previous week. Most of the time I was a pound or two lower. So things looked real good for this month.

2)   My change in weight from the previous day was starting to show some trends. Every Friday my weight would go up from Thursday, and every Thursday my weight would go down compared to Wednesday. Also every Tuesday, my weight would be less than Monday.

My Weight Graph for January

January Weight Chart

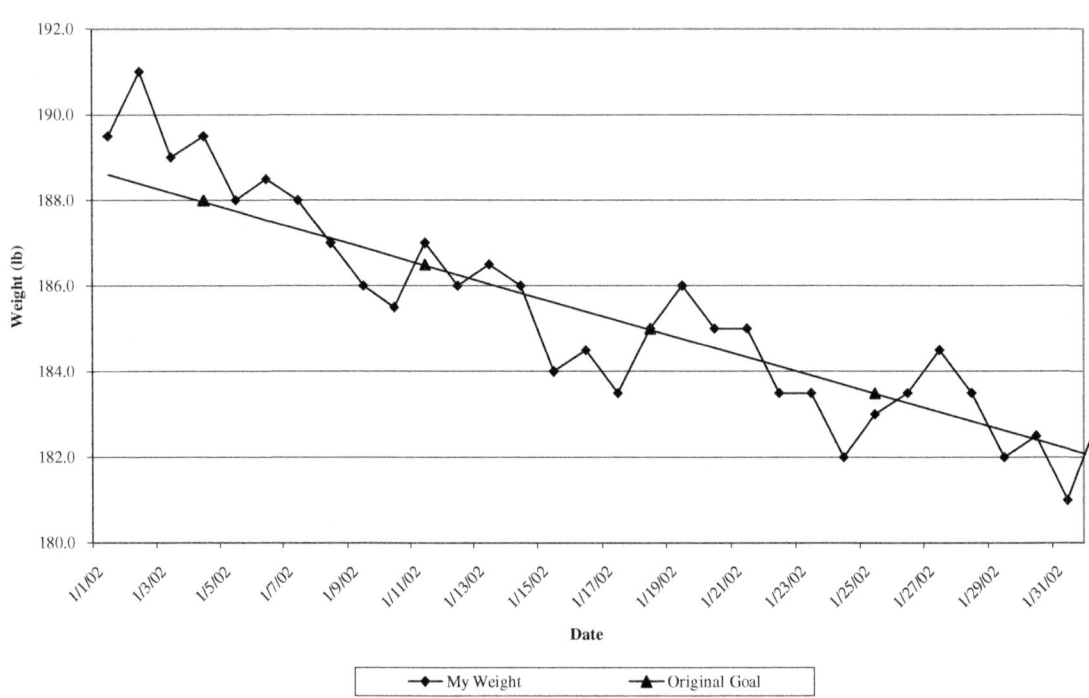

The graph of my weight in January looks fairly good. My weight line is basically following the goal line. Now the weight line bounced up and down and all around the goal line, which is expected and should happen. Weight loss is not a smooth process. When looking at the chart, I did not focus on a week; but I looked at a week compared to two or more weeks away from it. The group of points showed me if I was down in weight from a couple of weeks ago. I also needed to watch if the data trends continue with the weight loss from one day of the week to the other. Therefore, the January data proved the diet was going well.

A summary of my January analysis

Analyze

1. Some day to day trends are starting to appear.

2. Weight loss is going as planned.

Improve

1. No improvements needed.

My Weight Data for February

Date	Day of Week	Weight (lb)	Previous Day Change	Previous Week Change	1½ Pound Loss Goal
1-Feb-02	Friday	**183.0**	**2.0**	**0.0**	**182**
2-Feb-02	Saturday	184.0	1.0	0.5	
3-Feb-02	Sunday	182.0	(2.0)	(2.5)	
4-Feb-02	Monday	182.5	0.5	(1.0)	
5-Feb-02	Tuesday	180.0	(2.5)	(2.0)	
6-Feb-02	Wednesday	181.0	1.0	(1.5)	
7-Feb-02	Thursday	179.0	(2.0)	(2.0)	
8-Feb-02	Friday	**179.5**	**0.5**	**(3.5)**	**180.5**
9-Feb-02	Saturday	181.0	1.5	(3.0)	
10-Feb-02	Sunday	181.5	0.5	(0.5)	
11-Feb-02	Monday	181.5	0.0	(1.0)	
12-Feb-02	Tuesday	180.5	(1.0)	0.5	
13-Feb-02	Wednesday	180.0	(0.5)	(1.0)	
14-Feb-02	Thursday	179.0	(1.0)	0.0	
15-Feb-02	Friday	**179.5**	**0.5**	**0.0**	**179**
16-Feb-02	Saturday	181.0	1.5	0.0	
17-Feb-02	Sunday	182.0	1.0	0.5	
18-Feb-02	Monday	182.5	0.5	1.0	
19-Feb-02	Tuesday	180.0	(2.5)	(0.5)	
20-Feb-02	Wednesday	178.5	(1.5)	(1.5)	
21-Feb-02	Thursday	176.5	(2.0)	(2.5)	
22-Feb-02	Friday	**177.5**	**1.0**	**(2.0)**	**177.5**
23-Feb-02	Saturday	179.0	1.5	(2.0)	
24-Feb-02	Sunday	180.0	1.0	(2.0)	
25-Feb-02	Monday	178.5	(1.5)	(4.0)	
26-Feb-02	Tuesday	178.0	(0.5)	(2.0)	
27-Feb-02	Wednesday	179.0	1.0	0.5	
28-Feb-02	Thursday	177.5	(1.5)	1.0	
01-Mar-02	Friday	**176.5**	**(1.0)**	**(1.0)**	**176**

My observations from the February data are

1)   The weight loss was still meeting the goal line. I started the month at 183 pounds and ended the month at 176.5 pounds.

2)   The Tuesday, Thursday, and Friday day to day weight loss trends noticed in January continued in February.

3)   Every Saturday and Sunday, my weight would go up from the previous day.

My Weight Graph for February

February Weight Chart

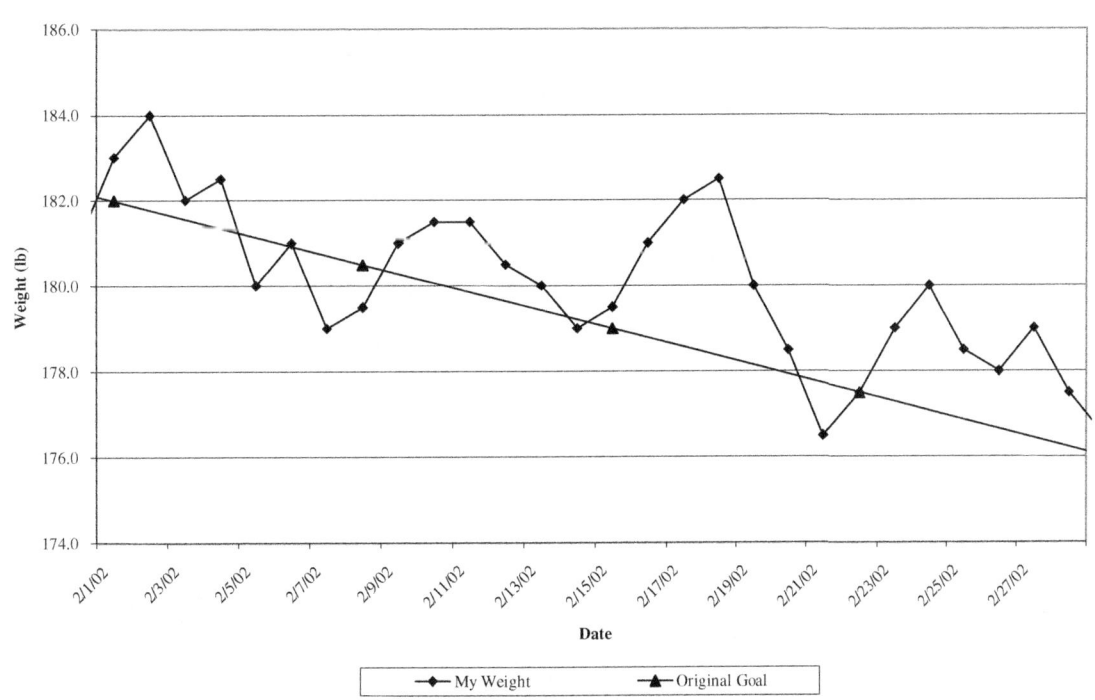

The weight line looked okay except for a big shoot up and drop at the end of the month. Otherwise, the data was following the same pattern.

I had enough information to look at why these things were happening. First, the spike and drop in weight at the end of February coincided with my daughter's birthday. I like birthday dinners with cake and ice cream, and it showed on the graph. The easiest day to day trend to explain was my weight drop every Thursday. I played basketball every Wednesday night. As a result, I would lose weight due to burning off all of my calories, and I would show some weight loss due to water loss. So then on Friday, I increased in weight due mostly to getting enough water in my body. I wondered if I was really losing weight due to basketball. I then looked at my Wednesday weight and compared it to Friday's weight. Sure enough, my Friday weight was always less than my Wednesday weight. Therefore, playing basketball was important in my diet. It looks like I will need to exercise to lose weight. I had always heard that in diet plans, but here I proved it with my weight chart.

Therefore, I had an explanation for Thursday and Friday, but what about Tuesday, Saturday, and Sunday? These three days were all connected. To explain, I have to analyze my eating habits. Friday nights and Saturdays are the days when my family eats out. During the week, I rarely eat out, and I do not eat big meals. So on Saturday and Sunday, my weight would go up due to eating out. Then on Tuesday, my body would recover from the weekend and show a weight loss.

From these observations, I learned a lot about my diet plan and myself. A summary of these observations are

1) Exercise is important, and I must keep exercising by continuing with basketball or exercise in another manner.

2) Eating out adversely affects my weight. If I eat out, I need to watch what I eat and watch the size of my portions of food.

3) Beware of birthday dinners and birthday parties with cake and ice cream.

A summary of my February analysis

Analyze

1. Exercising is important.
2. Eating out affects my weight loss.

Improve

1. Continue with exercising.
2. Eat carefully when eating out.

My Weight Data for March

Date	Day of Week	Weight (lb)	Previous Day Change	Previous Week Change	1½ Pound Loss Goal
1-Mar-02	Friday	**176.5**	**(1.0)**	**(1.0)**	**176**
2-Mar-02	Saturday	178.0	1.5	(1.0)	
3-Mar-02	Sunday	178.0	0.0	(2.0)	
4-Mar-02	Monday	178.5	0.5	0.0	
5-Mar-02	Tuesday	176.0	(2.5)	(2.0)	
6-Mar-02	Wednesday	177.5	1.5	(1.5)	
7-Mar-02	Thursday	175.5	(2.0)	(2.0)	
8-Mar-02	Friday	**177.0**	**1.5**	**0.5**	**174.5**
9-Mar-02	Saturday	179.0	2.0	1.0	
10-Mar-02	Sunday	178.5	(0.5)	0.5	
11-Mar-02	Monday	178.0	(0.5)	(0.5)	
12-Mar-02	Tuesday	177.5	(0.5)	1.5	
13-Mar-02	Wednesday	177.0	(0.5)	(0.5)	
14-Mar-02	Thursday	176.0	(1.0)	0.5	
15-Mar-02	Friday	**176.5**	**0.5**	**(0.5)**	**173**
16-Mar-02	Saturday	176.0	(0.5)	(3.0)	
17-Mar-02	Sunday	177.0	1.0	(1.5)	
18-Mar-02	Monday	177.0	0.0	(1.0)	
19-Mar-02	Tuesday	177.0	0.0	(0.5)	
20-Mar-02	Wednesday	177.0	0.0	0.0	
21-Mar-02	Thursday	175.0	(2.0)	(1.0)	
22-Mar-02	Friday	**176.5**	**1.5**	**0.0**	**171.5**
23-Mar-02	Saturday	175.5	(1.0)	(0.5)	
24-Mar-02	Sunday	174.5	(1.0)	(2.5)	
25-Mar-02	Monday	176.5	2.0	(0.5)	
26-Mar-02	Tuesday	176.0	(0.5)	(1.0)	
27-Mar-02	Wednesday	175.5	(0.5)	(1.5)	
28-Mar-02	Thursday	175.0	(0.5)	0.0	
29-Mar-02	Friday	**175.5**	**0.5**	**(1.0)**	**170**
30-Mar-02	Saturday	176.0	0.5	0.5	
31-Mar-02	Sunday	176.5	0.5	2.0	

My observations from the March data are

1) I started the month at 176.5 pounds, and I ended the month at 175.5 pounds; consequently, I only lost 1 pound during this month.

2) My weight basically stayed constant. I continued to lose weight from Wednesday night basketball, but this just made up for the rest of the week.

My Weight Graph for March

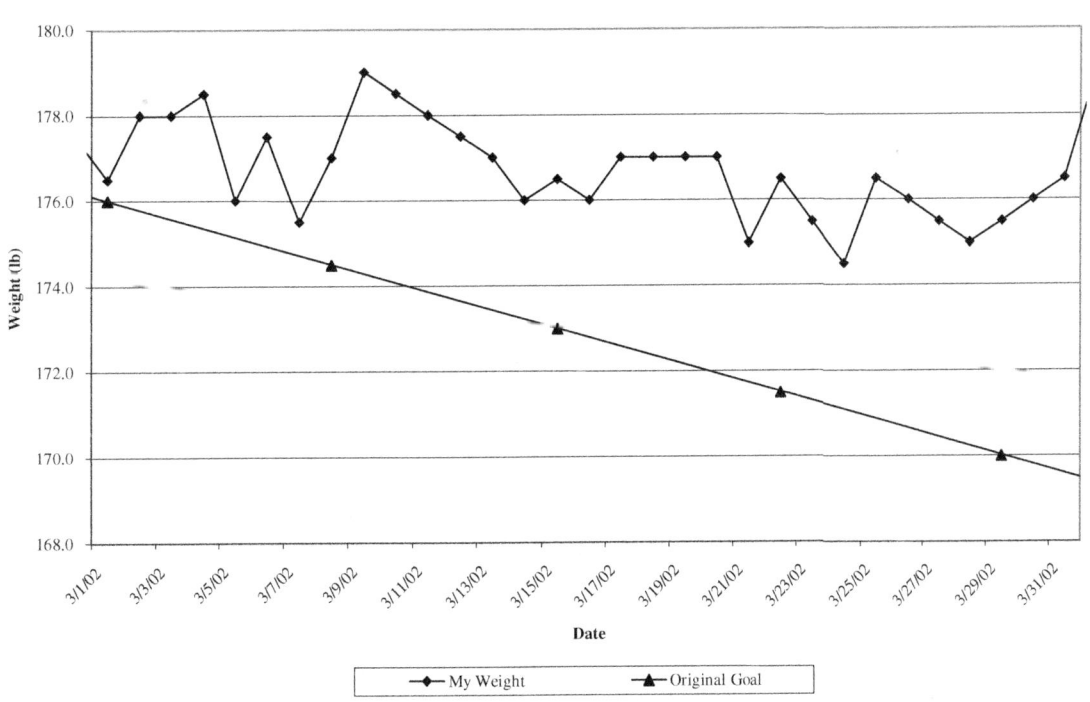

March Weight Chart

After following my 1½ pound weight loss per week goal line for January and February, I was obviously far away from this goal line by looking at the graph. I ended the month 5½ pounds above this goal, and I had a couple of concerns. One is why did I stay relatively flat in March, and what was I going to do about a goal line?

First, why did I not lose weight during March? Birthday parties were my big undoing in March. Not only is my birthday in March but also half of my family. So every week there was at least one big birthday dinner with cake and ice cream. I could not resist cake and ice cream.

However, I was doing everything else right during the week to lose my 1½ pounds a week, but the one or two birthday dinners covered it up. I also spent three days sitting in a chair watching the Big Ten college basketball tournament, so I just sat and ate while watching nine games in three days. This did not do me any favors either.

I needed a goal line to keep myself on track, but the goal line I had was pretty much unattainable. So what did I do? In my case, I kept my 1½ pound goal line on my graph to show my original plan. I went back to my original wager, which was to lose 20 pounds in 5 months. To reach that goal, I needed to lose 1 pound a week. I went back to my graph and added a goal line of 1 pound per week. Fortunately, my weight was right at the goal line of 1 pound per week, and so I used this as my new goal line. I wanted to keep my weight between the two goal lines.

My Weight Graph for March with 1 Pound Loss Goal Line Added

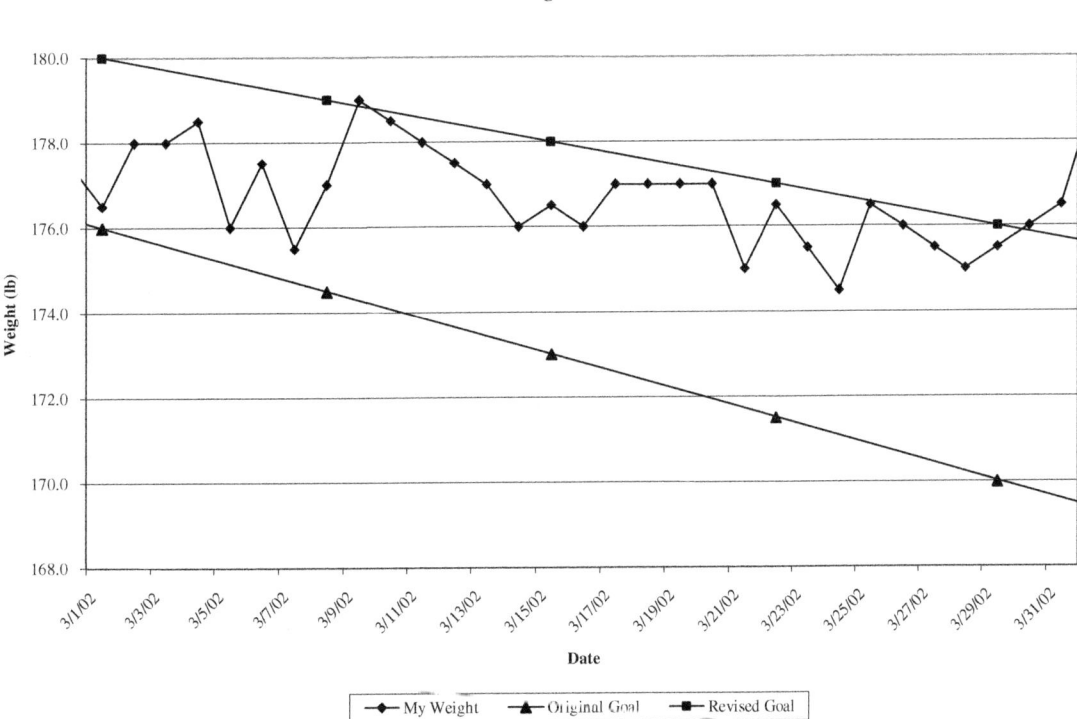

March Weight Chart

I think revising my goal line was an important decision for me. If I did not restate my goal line, my goal would be basically unattainable which would have lead me to ignore it. This would, in essence, leave me with no goals. If one does not have a goal, one cannot get to where he/she is going.

Therefore, if one gets off his/her goal line for weight loss by an amount one realistically cannot get back to, then he/she should restate his/her goals. I left my original goal as a reference, but I started following my new goal. This kept me going down my path of weight loss. One should not be afraid to restate one's goal because if his/her goals are meaningless, then he/she really does not have a goal.

Therefore, I learned the following things from my experiences in March:

1) Birthday parties are bad for my diet, and I need to come up with a moderation or substitution plan for the next batch of birthday parties. Most likely, I will need to concentrate on eating in moderation.

2) There are going to be special events that go over a few days or a week. If I cannot lose weight during these events, I need to try to manage myself so I do not add weight. I need to try at a minimum to just stay even on weight.

3) Having goals or a goal line is essential. If I fall off the goal line to the point that it is meaningless or unattainable, I restate my goals. If I do not restate my goals, then I do not have a true goal; and I will be worse off than if I restated them. I must always have realistic goals and goal line so that I can keep myself on track.

A summary of my March analysis

Analyze

1. Birthday parties adversely affect my weight.

2. Special events adversely affect my weight.

3. Restate the goal if the current goal is unattainable.

Improve

1. Eat in moderation at birthday parties.

2. Do the best I can at special events.

3. Restate the new goal.

My Weight Data for April

Date	Day of Week	Weight (lb)	Previous Day Change	Previous Week Change	1½ Pound Loss Goal	1 Pound Loss Goal
1-Apr-02	Monday	179.0	2.5	2.5		
2-Apr-02	Tuesday	177.0	(2.0)	1.0		
3-Apr-02	Wednesday	176.0	(1.0)	0.5		
4-Apr-02	Thursday	175.5	(0.5)	0.5		
5-Apr-02	Friday	**175.0**	**(0.5)**	**(0.5)**	**168.5**	**175**
6-Apr-02	Saturday	177.0	2.0	1.0		
7-Apr-02	Sunday	175.0	(2.0)	(1.5)		
8-Apr-02	Monday	175.5	0.5	(3.5)		
9-Apr-02	Tuesday	174.5	(1.0)	(2.5)		
10-Apr-02	Wednesday	173.5	(1.0)	(2.5)		
11-Apr-02	Thursday	171.0	(2.5)	(4.5)		
12-Apr-02	Friday	**171.5**	**0.5**	**(3.5)**	**167**	**174**
13-Apr-02	Saturday	173.0	1.5	(4.0)		
14-Apr-02	Sunday	175.0	2.0	0.0		
15-Apr-02	Monday	173.0	(2.0)	(2.5)		
16-Apr-02	Tuesday	172.0	(1.0)	(2.5)		
17-Apr-02	Wednesday	171.5	(0.5)	(2.0)		
18-Apr-02	Thursday	171.5	0.0	0.5		
19-Apr-02	Friday	**173.0**	**1.5**	**1.5**	**165.5**	**173**
20-Apr-02	Saturday	173.5	0.5	0.5		
21-Apr-02	Sunday	173.5	0.0	(1.5)		
22-Apr-02	Monday	173.0	(0.5)	0.0		
23-Apr-02	Tuesday	172.5	(0.5)	0.5		
24-Apr-02	Wednesday	171.0	(1.5)	(0.5)		
25-Apr-02	Thursday	170.0	(1.0)	(1.5)		
26-Apr-02	Friday	**171.0**	**1.0**	**(2.0)**	**164**	**172**
27-Apr-02	Saturday	173.0	2.0	(0.5)		
28-Apr-02	Sunday	173.5	0.5	0.0		
29-Apr-02	Monday	172.5	(1.0)	(0.5)		
30-Apr-02	Tuesday	170.5	(2.0)	(2.0)		

My observations from the April data are

1)   I started the month at 175.0 pounds, and I went down to 170.0 pounds at the end of the month. I was able to slightly exceed my revised weight plan loss of 1 pound per week.

2)   The trends continued of losing weight after basketball night and adding some weight over the weekend.

My Weight Graph for April

April Weight Chart

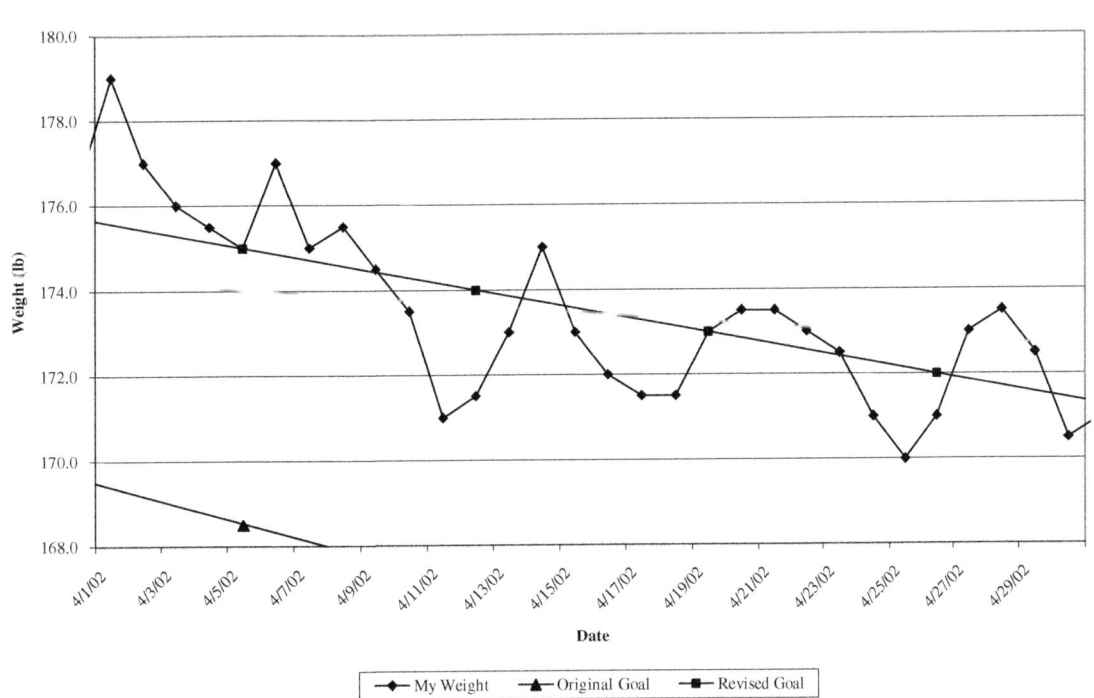

The weight line followed the goal line of 1 pound lost per week. There were definite fluctuations in the weight line, but it was drifting down along the 1 pound per week goal line.

After having a flat month in March, it looked like I was back on track. I was not losing 1½ pounds a week like I originally was able to obtain, but I was losing my revised goal of 1 pound per week.

A summary of my April analysis

Analyze

1. Trends of previous months except for March are continuing.

2. I am able to achieve the revised goal of 1 pound lost per week.

Improve

1. Everything looks fine, so there are no new improvement actions to take.

My Weight Data for May

Date	Day of Week	Weight (lb)	Previous Day Change	Previous Week Change	1½ Pound Loss Goal	1 Pound Loss Goal
1-May-02	Wednesday	171.0	0.5	0.0		
2-May-02	Thursday	169.5	(1.5)	(0.5)		
3-May-02	Friday	**170.0**	**0.5**	**(1.0)**	**162.5**	**171**
4-May-02	Saturday	169.0	(1.0)	(4.0)		
5-May-02	Sunday	170.0	1.0	(3.5)		
6-May-02	Monday	171.0	1.0	(1.5)		
7-May-02	Tuesday	170.0	(1.0)	(0.5)		
8-May-02	Wednesday	169.5	(0.5)	(1.5)		
9-May-02	Thursday	167.5	(2.0)	(2.0)		
10-May-02	Friday	**169.0**	**1.5**	**(1.0)**	**161**	**170**
11-May-02	Saturday	169.0	0.0	0.0		
12-May-02	Sunday	169.0	0.0	(1.0)		
13-May-02	Monday	171.0	2.0	0.0		
14-May-02	Tuesday	169.5	(1.5)	(0.5)		
15-May-02	Wednesday	169.0	(0.5)	(0.5)		
16-May-02	Thursday	166.0	(3.0)	(1.5)		
17-May-02	Friday	**168.0**	**2.0**	**(1.0)**	**161**	**169**
18-May-02	Saturday	168.0	0.0	(1.0)		
19-May-02	Sunday	169.5	1.5	0.5		
20-May-02	Monday	168.5	(1.0)	(2.5)		
21-May-02	Tuesday	167.5	(1.0)	(2.0)		
22-May-02	Wednesday	167.5	0.0	(1.5)		
23-May-02	Thursday	164.5	(3.0)	(1.5)		
24-May-02	Friday	**166.5**	**2.0**	**(1.5)**	**161**	**168**
25-May-02	Saturday	167.0	0.5	(1.0)		
26-May-02	Sunday	167.0	0.0	(2.5)		
27-May-02	Monday	168.0	1.0	(0.5)		
28-May-02	Tuesday	168.5	0.5	1.0		
29-May-02	Wednesday	168.0	(0.5)	0.5		
30-May-02	Thursday	165.0	(3.0)	0.5		
31-May-02	Friday	**166.5**	**1.5**	**0.0**	**161**	**167**

My observations from the May weight data are

1) I started the month at 170.0 pounds, and I ended the month at 166.5 pounds. I lost 1 or 1½ pounds a week the first 3 weeks, but I did not lose any weight the last week. This last week included Memorial Day, and I had two family gatherings that weekend.

2) Other than the last week, all other data looked like a continuation of the weight loss rate and daily trends.

My Weight Graph for May

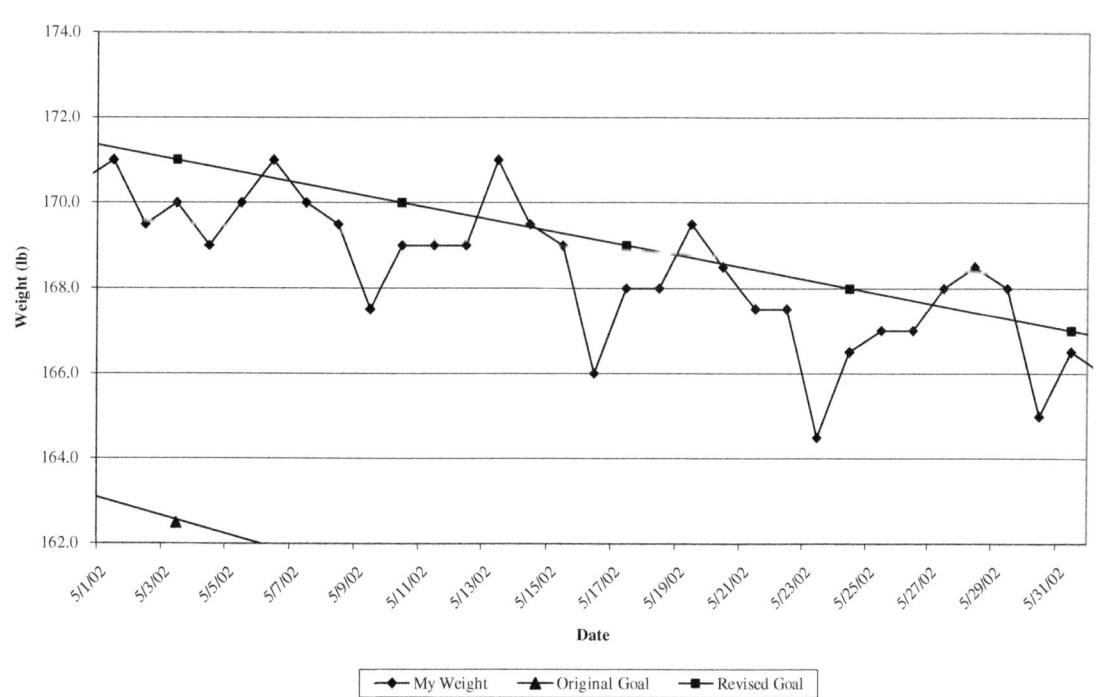

May Weight Chart

Even though there are some points above the weight goal line, most of the points are below the goal line. It appears that I am building separation between my weight and the goal line. There is no problem with this. This is helpful for when I have a no loss week. I am still able to meet the goal for the week because of the buffer.

Family gatherings once again caught me. This was a replay of the March birthday parties syndrome. I was not able to lose weight the Memorial Day week, but I also did not gain any weight. Therefore, it was not good, but it also was not terrible. This is a situation where the weight buffer helped.

At this point in time, I reached my initial weight goal of 168 pounds. I then wondered if this was the right amount of weight for me or should it be different. I was thinking it should be lower based upon my high school weight, but I did not know what it should be.

Fortunately for me, my company has a fitness center located on its campus. It has physical fitness personnel who helped me with this question. It might also be good to consult one's personal physician.

There were two ways that I could have gotten this information from them. One was for them to look up in a table what a normal person should weigh. The other choice was for them to do body fat measurements on me to determine my body fat percentage. I chose the more accurate route of body fat measurements.

After completion of the measurements and doing the calculations, they determined that my target weight should be 163 pounds. I used this weight as my new goal weight. I then set my goal to reach 161 pounds. I did this to assure myself that once I reached my target weight, I would stay below or at this target weight.

A summary of my May analysis

Analyze

1. Family gatherings are still my enemy. I am not able to eat in moderation so that I will not over do it.
2. My normal eating routine is continuing to work.

Improve

1. At the next family gathering, I need to fill my stomach with something low in calories so that I will be better able to eat in moderation.
2. There is no need to adjust my normal eating routine since the weight loss is meeting the goal.
3. Revise the final weight goal from 168 pounds to 161 pounds.

My Weight Data for June

Date	Day of Week	Weight (lb)	Previous Day Change	Previous Week Change	1½ Pound Loss Goal	1 Pound Loss Goal
1-Jun-02	Saturday	166.0	(0.5)	(1.0)		
2-Jun-02	Sunday	167.0	1.0	0.0		
3-Jun-02	Monday	166.0	(1.0)	(2.0)		
4-Jun-02	Tuesday	168.0	2.0	(0.5)		
5-Jun-02	Wednesday	167.0	(1.0)	(1.0)		
6-Jun-02	Thursday	167.5	0.5	2.5		
7-Jun-02	Friday	**166.5**	**(1.0)**	**0.0**	**161**	**166**
8-Jun-02	Saturday	166.5	0.0	0.5		
9-Jun-02	Sunday	166.5	0.0	(0.5)		
10-Jun-02	Monday	167.0	0.5	1.0		
11-Jun-02	Tuesday	167.0	0.0	(1.0)		
12-Jun-02	Wednesday	167.5	0.5	0.5		
13-Jun-02	Thursday	167.5	0.0	0.0		
14-Jun-02	Friday	**167.5**	**0.0**	**1.0**	**161**	**165**
15-Jun-02	Saturday	168.0	0.5	1.5		
16-Jun-02	Sunday	168.0	0.0	1.5		
17-Jun-02	Monday	168.0	0.0	1.0		
18-Jun-02	Tuesday	166.5	(1.5)	(0.5)		
19-Jun-02	Wednesday	167.0	0.5	(0.5)		
20-Jun-02	Thursday	167.5	0.5	0.0		
21-Jun-02	Friday	**165.0**	**(2.5)**	**(2.5)**	**161**	**164**
22-Jun-02	Saturday	165.0	0.0	(3.0)		
23-Jun-02	Sunday	165.0	0.0	(3.0)		
24-Jun-02	Monday	166.0	1.0	(2.0)		
25-Jun-02	Tuesday	168.0	2.0	1.5		
26-Jun-02	Wednesday	166.5	(1.5)	(0.5)		
27-Jun-02	Thursday	166.0	(0.5)	(1.5)		
28-Jun-02	Friday	**165.0**	**(1.0)**	**0.0**	**161**	**163**
29-Jun-02	Saturday	165.0	0.0	0.0		
30-Jun-02	Sunday	166.5	1.5	1.5		

My observations from my June data are

1)   I started the month at 166.0 pounds, and I ended the month at 165.0 pounds. I only lost 1 pound during the entire month.

2)   I had changes in what I was doing this month. A couple of things happened. First, Wednesday night basketball ended and it would not begin again until September. Second, I went on vacation for a couple of weeks. For ten days, I did not take any weight measurements. This was from June 8 to June 16.

Note: I added the data for these dates by taking the June 7 reading and the June 17 reading and added weight measurements that represent a line between these two dates.

My Weight Graph for June

June Weight Chart

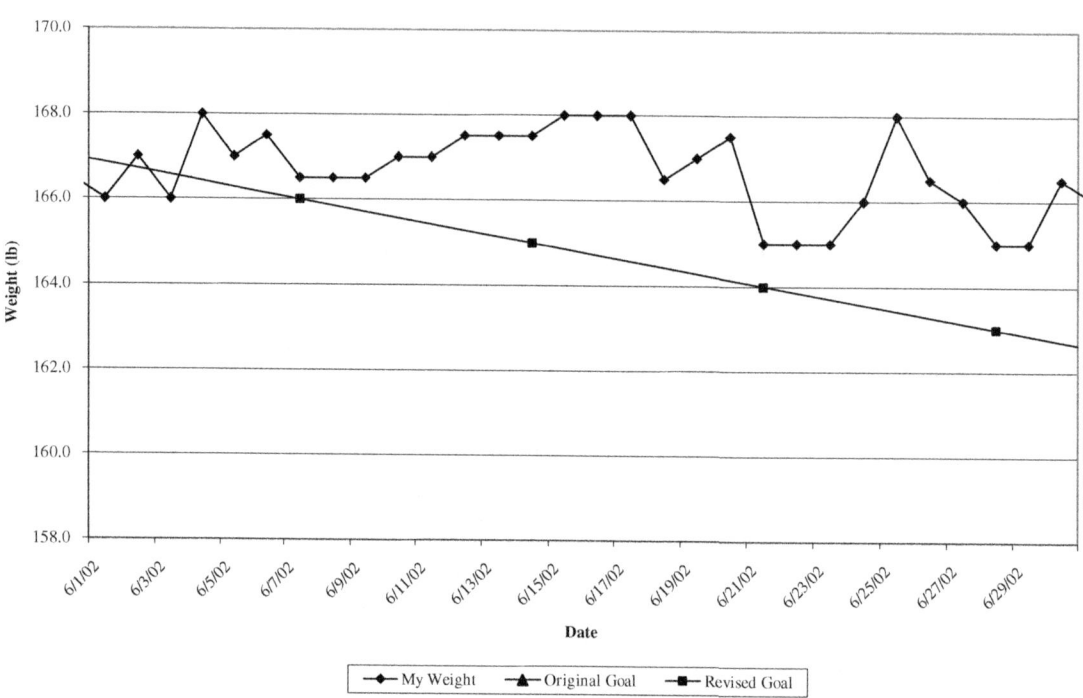

Vacations and my taking a break from strictly following my diet really showed on the graph. I was not diligent in my diet; I had many nighttime snacks and did not eat in moderation.

I definitely had to get back to following my diet. I did not see the need to restate my goal line because I was only a few pounds over the goal line. If I followed the diet, I should be able to slowly get back to the goal line. I did not have any real special events to stop me from losing weight. I basically went on vacation and took my diet on vacation, too.

A summary of my June analysis

Analyze

1. I did not follow my diet plan because I had many snacks and did not eat in moderation.

2. I am not far enough away from my goal line to have to restate the goal line.

Improve

1. I must get back to following my diet plan.

My Weight Data for July

Date	Day of Week	Weight (lb)	Previous Day Change	Previous Week Change	1½ Pound Loss Goal	1 Pound Loss Goal
1-Jul-02	Monday	166.0	(0.5)	0.0		
2-Jul-02	Tuesday	165.0	(1.0)	(3.0)		
3-Jul-02	Wednesday	164.0	(1.0)	(2.5)		
4-Jul-02	Thursday	162.5	(1.5)	(3.5)		
5-Jul-02	Friday	**164.0**	**1.5**	**(1.0)**	**161**	**161**
6-Jul-02	Saturday	164.0	0.0	(1.0)		
7-Jul-02	Sunday	162.0	(2.0)	(4.5)		
8-Jul-02	Monday	161.5	(0.5)	(4.5)		
9-Jul-02	Tuesday	161.5	0.0	(3.5)		
10-Jul-02	Wednesday	163.5	2.0	(0.5)		
11-Jul-02	Thursday	162.0	(1.5)	(0.5)		
12-Jul-02	Friday	**160.0**	**(2.0)**	**(4.0)**	**161**	**161**
13-Jul-02	Saturday	159.5	(0.5)	(4.5)		
14-Jul-02	Sunday	161.0	1.5	(1.0)		
15-Jul-02	Monday	160.0	(1.0)	(1.5)		
16-Jul-02	Tuesday	160.0	0.0	(1.5)		
17-Jul-02	Wednesday	160.5	0.5	(3.0)		
18-Jul-02	Thursday	161.0	0.5	(1.0)		
19-Jul-02	Friday	**161.5**	**0.5**	**1.5**	**161**	**161**
20-Jul-02	Saturday	161.5	0.0	2.0		
21-Jul-02	Sunday	162.0	0.5	1.0		
22-Jul-02	Monday	162.0	0.0	2.0		
23-Jul-02	Tuesday	162.5	0.5	2.5		
24-Jul-02	Wednesday	163.0	0.5	2.5		
25-Jul-02	Thursday	163.5	0.5	2.5		
26-Jul-02	Friday	**161.5**	**(2.0)**	**0.0**	**161**	**161**
27-Jul-02	Saturday	160.5	(1.0)	(1.0)		
28-Jul-02	Sunday	163.5	3.0	1.5		
29-Jul-02	Monday	164.5	1.0	2.5		
30-Jul-02	Tuesday	163.0	(1.5)	0.5		
31-Jul-02	Wednesday	161.0	(2.0)	(2.0)		

My observations from my July data are

1)   I started the month at 166.0 pounds, and I ended the month at 161.0 pounds. I was able to lose 5 pounds during this month.

2)   I had completed my diet to lose weight. I had a goal to reach 161 pounds. With me being at 161 pounds, I was officially calling my diet complete.

3)   I basically reached my weight goal in the middle of July. I had a week long trip during the middle of the month. I put on some weight during this week, so I spent a couple of weeks getting back down to 161 pounds.

My Weight Graph for July

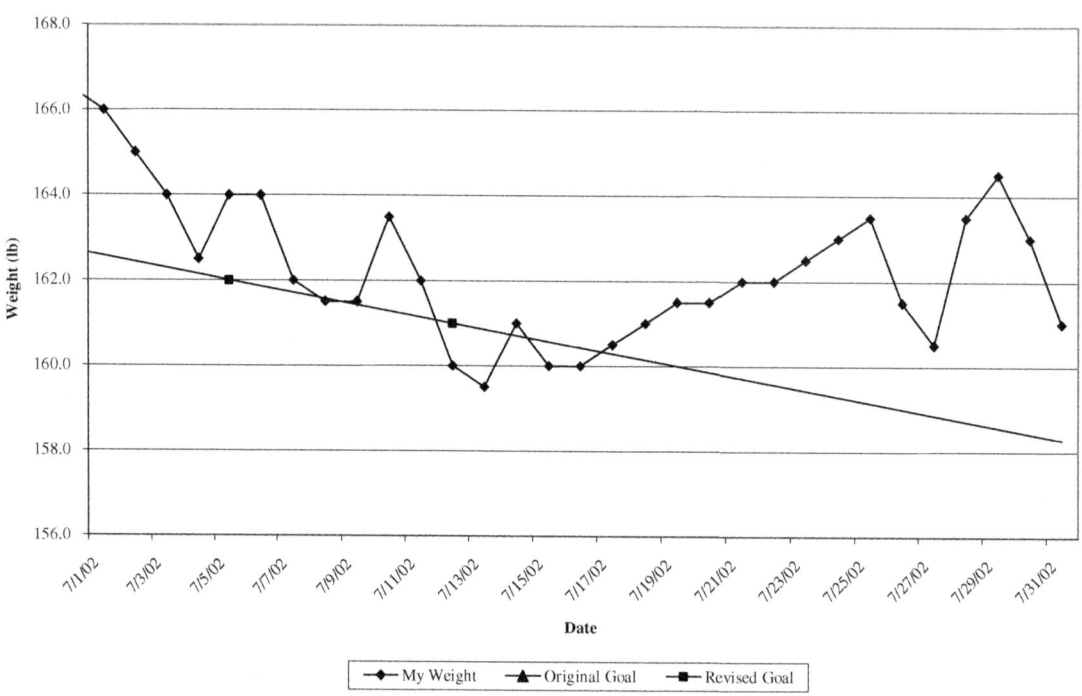

July Weight Chart

Vacations and trips once again got me for a few pounds. I will always need to be careful on trips not to overdo it too much. I will always probably gain weight on trips since they change my eating routine. I will need to remember this so that when I know a trip is coming up, I can start the trip with my weight on the low side to allow me more room to add a few pounds.

I also had the normal weight gain due to a family gathering. This appeared to be my other weak spot. Therefore, just like the trips, I will need to be aware of the family gatherings and try to be on the low side of my weight range.

A summary of my July analysis

Analyze

1. I continue to add some weight from trips and family gatherings.
2. I have reached my weight goal.

Improve

1. I have completed the Improve stage. I can proceed to the next stage.
2. I need to remember my lessons learned during this diet to assist me in the next stage when I need it.
3. I need not to go wild and start eating everything in sight because I will have to start right back on the diet. I need to keep my controlled eating habits, but now I can have a snack if I get real hungry. My food intake can go up but not too much.

By reaching my weight loss goal in July, I had completed the Analyze and Improve Phases of my Six Sigma weight loss plan.

To analyze the data, I looked for trends in the data. Did I lose weight consistently on a given day? Did special events affect the weight loss? Was the weight loss meeting the goals? I looked at the data and graph to find out what worked and what did not work. I basically ask the question: Am I losing weight like I expected? If yes, what is working for me? If no, why did it not go as expected?

In the Improve Phase, I addressed the basic question if the answer to the previous question was no. I looked for the root cause of the problem and then devised a way to fix this root cause.

In my case, family gatherings were my biggest root cause. One way to improve this would be not to go to family gatherings. This was not an acceptable solution, so I had to find another way. I first tried to eat in moderation, but I was unable to do that at first. I was able to eat in more moderation for the July 4th gatherings. I just had to really dedicate myself to eating in moderation at family gatherings.

I had another root cause for not losing weight, which was eating out. I addressed this by eating in moderation when possible or by substituting lower calorie food for high calorie food.

The Improve Phase also pointed out things I needed to continue to do. The two main things to continue were to play basketball or exercise and to follow my eating plan. I had to continue doing these two things while improving on my two major root causes.

The other thing I did was to keep a realistic goal for my weight loss. I had to revise my goals, and I was then able to keep this goal. It is okay to revise goals so that one actually has a goal. There is a limit, however, to how many times one should revise the goals. If one is revising goals all of the time, then he/she is not getting anywhere. One should go back and analyze why he/she is having problems and then come up with a true improvement plan that will address that problem. The goal should be revised due to special circumstances and not due to normal happenings. Normal happenings have to be addressed to make the weight loss plan work, though. Special circumstances are a bump in the road that sends one off course but are something that one can continue down the road after he/she gets past the bump.

The Control Phase

How many times has a person reached his/her weight goal and then one year later is back at the old weight? A big part of Six Sigma is to sustain what one has done. It is called "Sustain the Gain." In this case, however, it is "Sustain the Loss."

So how does a person sustain the loss? Basically this can be achieved through the use of a control chart. One question always is, if I put some weight back on, how much is too much? Another question is, how do I know when I am starting to get out of control? The control chart is made to answer these questions. It provides a great visual picture if things are going okay, and it tells when one is having a problem.

Therefore, for the Control Phase of my Six Sigma weight loss plan, I used a control chart. A control chart consists of two main items. The first item is the actual measurement made. This is nothing different from what one would be doing during the weight loss phase. Everyday I took a weight measurement, entered it into the data table, and then graphed the point.

One might ask, "Am I going to have to weigh myself everyday for years?" The answer is yes and no. One will need to take a weight measurement at some consistent time period. If things initially go real well during the Control Phase, then a person might be able to weigh every third day. I would not go beyond every fourth day because one may not know for a month if he/she is in control of his/her weight. To start off, one should continue to weigh everyday until one feels comfortable that he/she can weigh less frequently and still stay in control.

The second part of the control chart is the control lines. There are 3 lines: Desired Level (or middle point), Upper Limit, and Lower Limit. The desired level is the weight one wants to achieve and maintain. The upper and lower limits are lines that show how far one's weight can drift from the desired weight and still be statistically at the desired weight. As one will discover, one's weight never just stays at one weight level. A person's weight goes up and down during the day and between days.

My August Control Chart

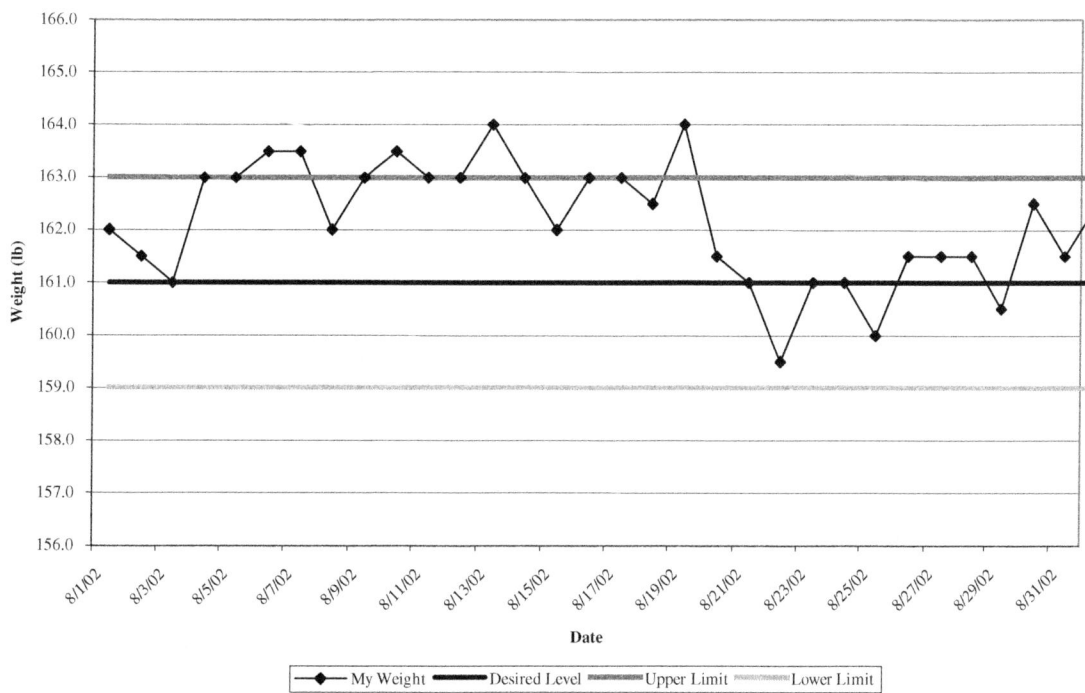

August Control Chart

How can one analyze a control chart? He/she should analyze the control chart by using these 3 rules:

1) Any measurement point above the upper limit or below the lower limit

2) Anytime that there are 7 measurements in a row between the upper limit line and desired level line or between the lower limit line and desired level line

3) Anytime that there are 7 measurements in a row that are going up or going down

Rule 1 Sample Control Chart

Point Above or Below the Limit Lines

Rule 1 Sample Control Chart

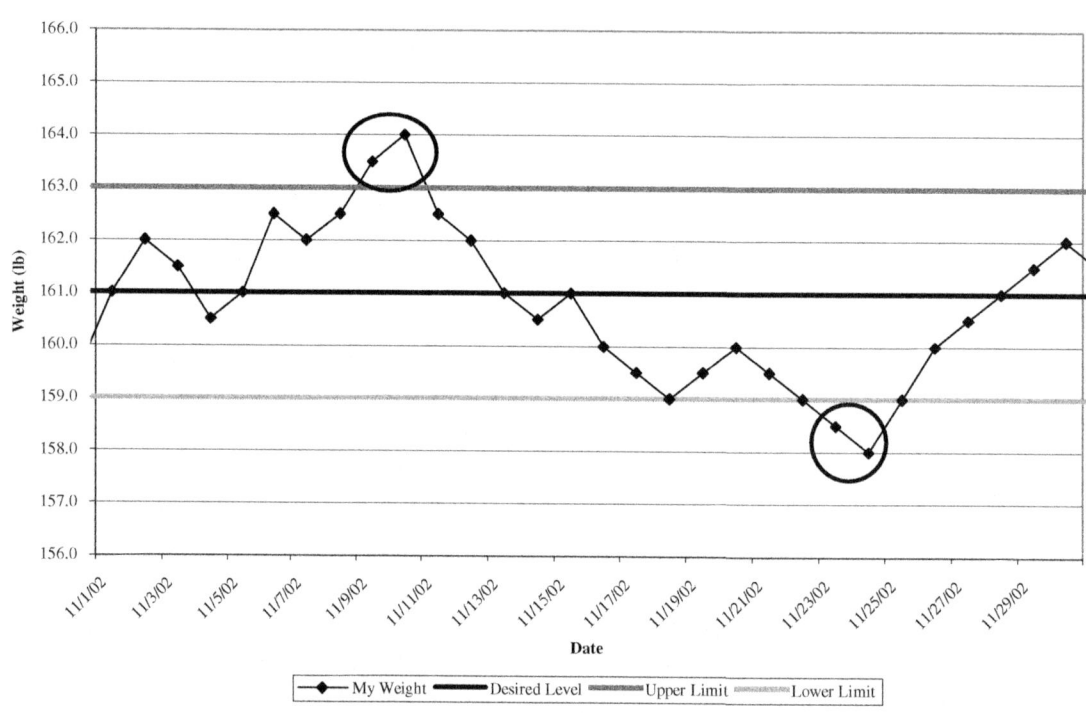

There are two areas where two points are out of control. These areas are circled on the graph. It only takes one measurement outside of the control limit to have the weight out of control.

Rule 2 Sample Control Chart

7 Points Above or Below Desired Level

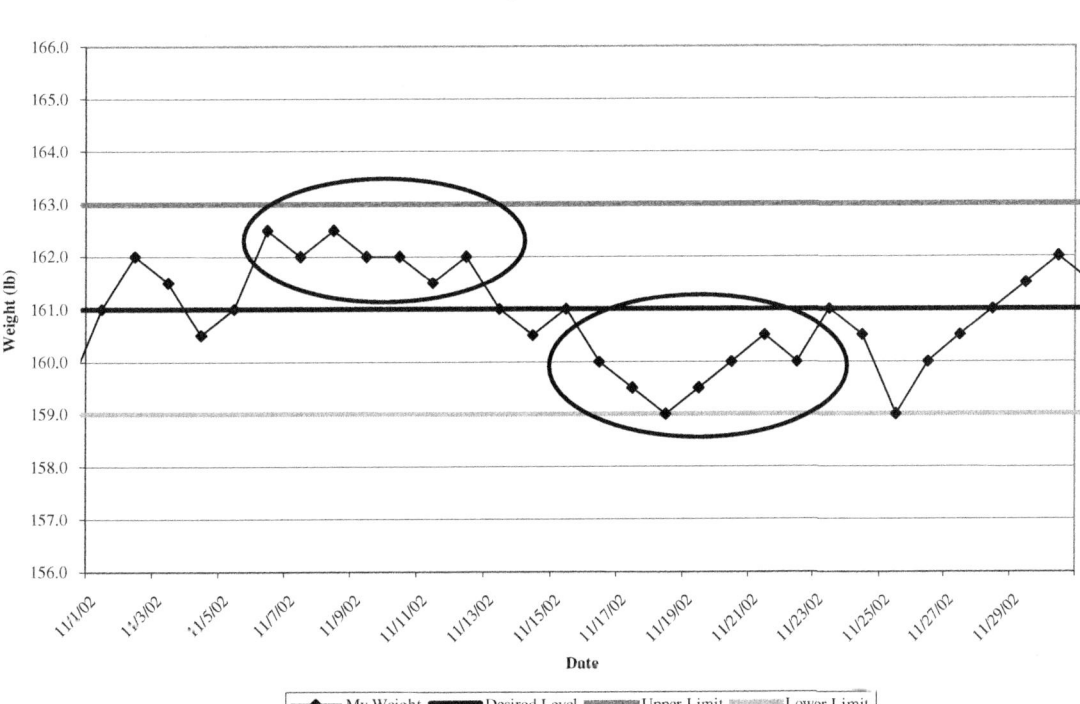

Rule 2 Sample Control Chart

There are two areas of the sample control chart that are out of control. These circled areas are situations when the control chart shows that one's weight is out of control. They are out of control because of the seven consecutive points below or above the desired level.

Rule 3 Sample Control Chart

7 Points in a Row Up or Down

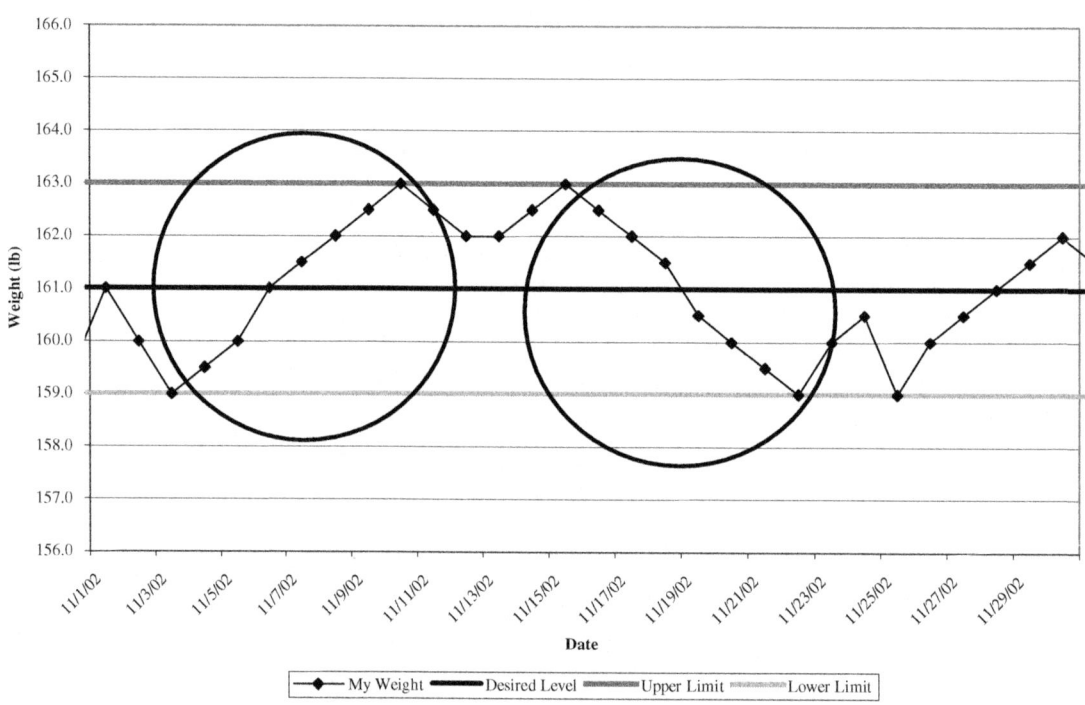

Rule 3 Sample Control Chart

Obviously, there are two parts of the sample graph that one had either 7 points in a row going up or down. When this shows up, a person knows that his/her weight is out of control.

A person can use a spreadsheet or graph paper to construct the control chart. The chart is very similar to the graph that would be used for the weight loss part of this book. The graph has the desired weight in the middle of the vertical axis. Drawing a line straight across at the desired weight is the midpoint for one's control chart.

Now one needs to add the upper and lower limit lines. The upper limit should be the desired weight plus 2 pounds, and the lower limit should be the desired weight minus 2 pounds. The difference between the desired level and the limit lines can be 3 pounds, however. From my experience, 2 pounds kept me in good control. The goal is for a person to keep his/her weight at the desired level in the long run.

Therefore, the control chart should look something like this:

Sample Control Chart

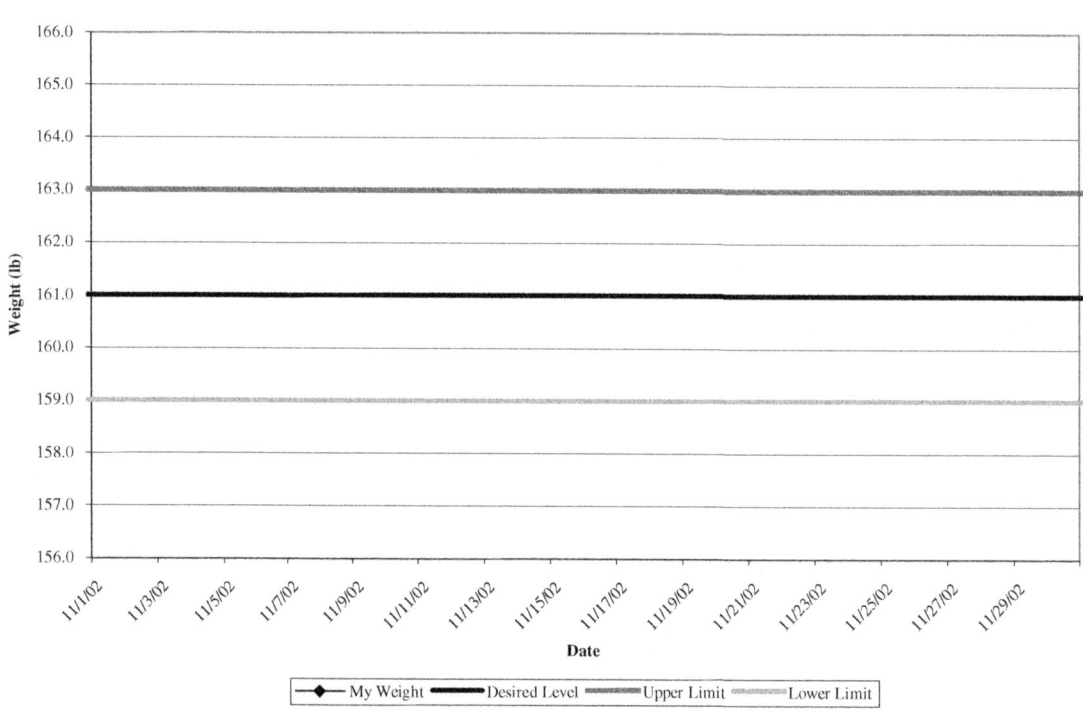

Sample Control Chart

Now all one does is add his/her weight measurements to the control chart. The weight measurements should be done at regular intervals. If one misses a weight measurement, he/she should continue on and skip that reading on the control chart.

To analyze the control chart, one should just utilize the three rules. When a person has a time when his/her weight is out of control, he/she can analyze why that is happening. Was there a special event? Have eating habits changed during that time? One has to try to figure out what happened during the time the weight went out of control and figure out an improvement action to get the weight back into control.

Once out of control, one must attempt to get back in control as soon as possible. One may have to go back on the diet if he/she is above the upper control limit. The longer one waits to get back into control, the harder and longer it will take to get back to where he/she wants to be.

Therefore, if one uses the control chart process, he/she should be able to keep his/her weight at the desired level and not have to start another diet a year from now. This is the real power of Six Sigma. Once one reaches the goal, he/she should stay at that goal.

My Weight Control Chart for August

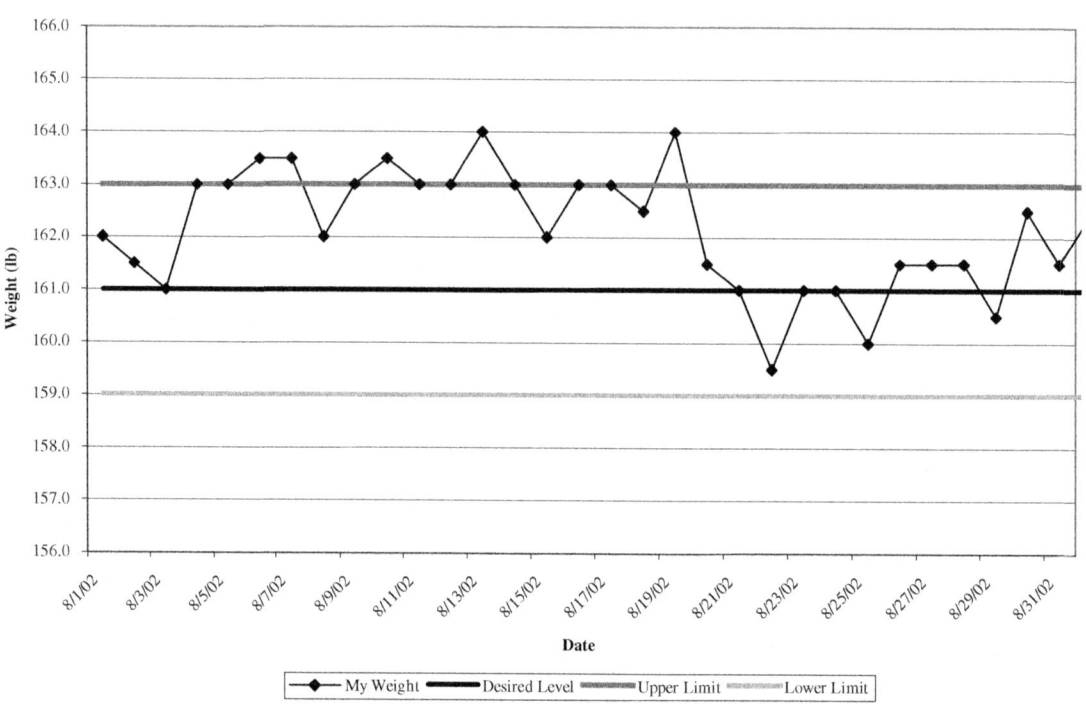

August Control Chart

For example, I was out of control for most of the month of August. From August 4 to August 20, I was really out of control. I had 5 points that were above the upper limit.

After August 20, I was back in control. Consequently, I was able to get my out of control weight back under control. I was able to get back in control by doing the things I did while I was dieting. I did not have to go strictly by the diet, but I did some of the basic things to lose the weight I needed to get back in control.

The control chart worked well for me because it showed me right away that I was putting too much weight back on. It helped me stop the bad habits before I got too far from my target weight. I fell in the trap, as most everyone does, of going back to eating and putting some pounds back on. After two weeks of going out of control, I was able to get back to my goal.

If I used a 3 pound range instead of the 2 pound range on my control chart, I still would have been out of control. I would have had 7 or more points between the upper limit and the desired level.

Therefore, by analyzing my control chart, I was able to keep my weight in control by making changes when my weight began moving upward. Every time one's weight goes out of control, he/she needs to analyze why and make the appropriate improvement action.

My Weight Control Chart for September and October

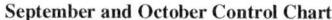

September and October Control Chart

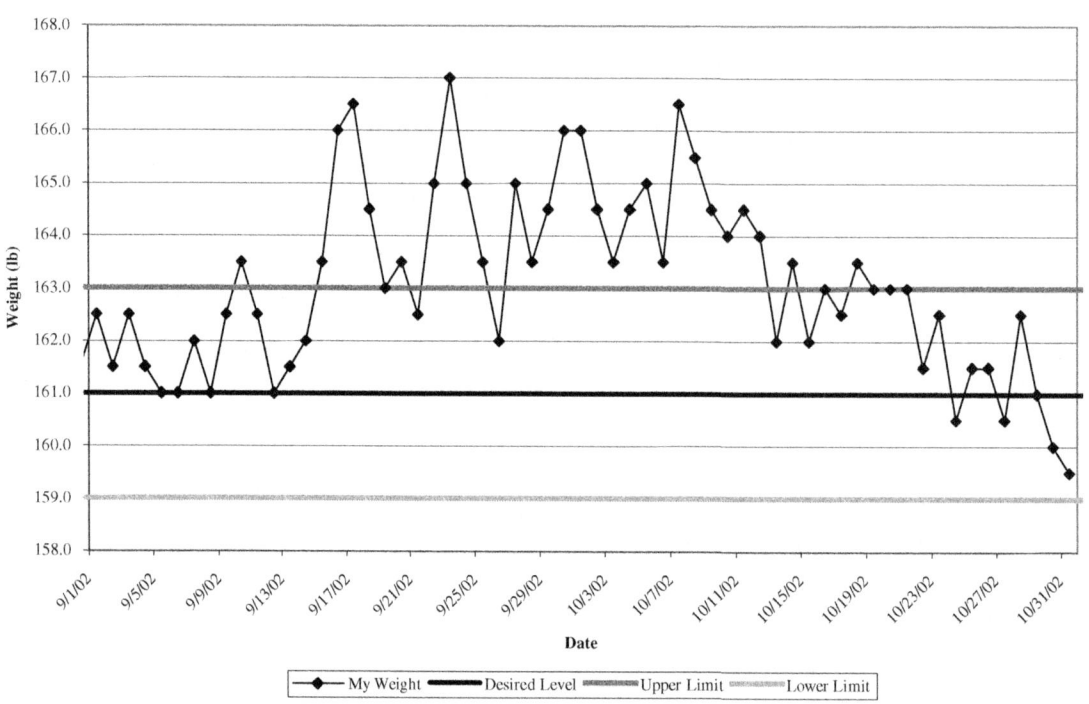

The control chart for September and October has three distinct areas. During the first part of September, my weight was in control. Then from mid-September to mid-October, my weight was clearly out of control. Finally, during the last part of October, I was able to get my weight back into control.

In the first part of September, I was in control of my weight per the control chart rules. I had a warning sign in the control chart because I did not have any weight measurements below 161 pounds. I was in control, but I could easily go out of control.

Unfortunately, this came true from mid-September to mid-October. I went way out of control. I even got to 6 pounds over my desired weight. I let myself go, and I did not get my weight back down.

If I moved my desired weight up 4 pounds to 165 pounds and did the same for my upper and lower limits, my weight was actually in control between 163 pounds and 167 pounds. Clearly, weight can be in control even if it is not at the wanted desired level.

After one month of being out of control, I began to wonder if I just wanted to stay at this weight range, or did I want to make myself get back down to my desired level. I decided that I worked too hard to just give up and control my weight at 165 pounds. What happens if my weight goes up again? Do I increase my desired weight level so that my weight is in control? This seems to be the start of a vicious cycle that I had already lived on my previous diets. Therefore, I had to get my weight back under control at 161 pounds. During the last part of October, I was able to once again get my weight under control at my desired weight of 161 pounds.

I know that this will not be the last time I go out of control, but I have been able to go out of control and still get back into control without too much suffering. Each time I get myself back into control, I am learning more about how I can stay in control.

I reviewed the three months of my control progress. During that time period, my weight went out of control two times. This is probably normal since I changed my eating habits and I had not learned how I could eat and stay in control. By working through two of the out of control times, I was able to learn more about how I could eat and be in control of my weight. In the future, I should have less occurrences of out of control weight as I continually learn about myself.

So once a person reaches the desired weight, he/she should start the Control Phase of Six Sigma. One can control his/her weight by using a control chart. By keeping the weight between the upper and lower control limits, one will effectively "Sustain the Loss" that he/she worked so hard to do. Following the control chart will keep a person from having to go on a diet again. To me, that makes the time to do the control chart worth every minute.

Six Sigma Applied to Other Things

This book has demonstrated how one can apply the Six Sigma business improvement program to weight loss. Six Sigma can be applied to other things, too. Anything that one can measure, he/she can apply Six Sigma to it.

A good example of this was a man who was recently diagnosed with diabetes. His diabetes was the milder Type 2 kind that can usually be controlled through diet and exercise. He created charts of his blood sugar levels. These charts helped him control his blood sugar level and enabled him to use diet and exercise to control his blood sugar level. He did not have to take the next step and start using insulin.

Another example could be to use this method in an athletic manner. In basketball, a person may want to increase his/her free throw percentage. One could track his/her free throw percentages in practices and see if he/she is actually making progress. It could also illustrate what helped the free throw percentage and what did not help it.

Therefore, one should not be intimidated by using the Six Sigma principles on something else in one's life. If there is something a person wants to change in life, he/she should try to measure it. Then through the measurements, one can analyze and improve what he/she would like to change. Then once the change is completed, one can keep it that way by controlling it. Realizing one's goals brings a great deal of satisfaction.

"Anything worth doing is worth doing well" is an old adage, but it still rings true today. Losing weight and keeping it off is a daily struggle, but feeling good, looking good, and enjoying good health make the struggle well worth it. Using Six Sigma makes it easier to achieve.

ISBN 155395437-8

9 781553 954378

Printed in Great Britain
by Amazon